Gold Standard Whey

Dr. Earl Rolfe

Whey

Whey, watery division that structures alongside curd when milk coagulates. It contains the water-solvent constituents of milk and is basically a 5 percent arrangement of lactose in water, for certain minerals and lactalbumin.

The whey is taken out from the curd during the method involved with making cheddar. Then it is centrifuged to eliminate fat, focused or dried, and utilized for food in handled cheddar items, baking, and candy making. Whey is utilized for creature feed as a fluid, concentrate, or dry powder.

Little Miss Muffet might have been well forward thinking. She was eating curds and whey before whey protein was a thing. Today, whey protein is a fixing in numerous dietary bars and shakes.

Enrolled dietitian Maxine Smith, RD, LD, makes sense of the advantages and disadvantages of whey protein and whether you really want this enhancement in your life.

What is whey protein?

Whey protein alludes to a gathering of eight proteins tracked down in milk. These proteins, all together from the greatest to littlest sums in milk, are:

- ✓ Beta-lacto globulin.
- ✓ Alpha-lactalbumin.
- ✓ Glycomacropeptide.
- ✓ Immunoglobulins.
- ✓ Ox-like serum egg whites.
- ✓ Lactoferrin.
- ✓ Lacto peroxidase.
- ✓ Lysozyme.

Producers add compounds to drain in the cheddar making process. The chemicals sour the milk, what isolates the fluid whey from milk's strong curds. The curds, which contain a large portion of the milk's fat, are the fundamental fixing in cheddar.

At the point when the strong curds are eliminated, you're left with watery whey protein, which has differing measures of lactose (milk sugar) and fat. As a rule, makers purify the whey to kill microbes and afterward dry it. Presto! Whey protein powder.

Kinds of whey protein

Whey protein then, at that point, goes through one more interaction to make one of three principal types:

Concentrate: Items with whey protein pack fluctuate broadly in their protein, lactose and fat substance. Whey protein pack is in numerous protein beverages, bars and healthful items. It's additionally utilized in newborn child equation.

Confine: This type is reliably high in protein and low in fat or lactose. You might see it recorded on the names of protein supplements, like bars and beverages. Whey protein detach might be a reasonable decision for individuals who are lactose prejudiced — however don't attempt any of these on the off chance that you have a milk sensitivity.

Hydrolysate: Otherwise called hydrolyzed whey protein, whey Hydrolysate is the simplest to process. It's delicate on processing on the grounds that its long protein chains, called peptides, are pre-separated into more limited ones. Specific baby equations frequently utilize hydrolyzed whey protein. You may likewise see it in clinical enhancements for nourishing lacks.

Amino acids and whey protein

Whey protein is a finished protein, containing every one of the nine fundamental amino acids. "Amino acids are significant for some capabilities in the body, from building muscle to making new safe cells," says Smith. Your body makes numerous amino acids all alone, yet not fundamental amino acids. You need to help fundamental amino acids through your eating routine, and consuming whey protein is one method for doing that. Yet, don't limit "fragmented" proteins. Most plant proteins, similar to vegetables and nuts, don't contain every one of the fundamental amino acids. Be that as it may, they have a lot of medical advantages. At the point when you eat various inadequate proteins, you get a sizable amount of fundamental amino acids to address your body's issues.

Advantages of whey protein

Muscle building: Muscles love protein, particularly complete proteins like whey. "Whey protein contains spread chain amino acids, a particular sort of amino corrosive that assists with muscle building," Smith says.

Wound recuperating: The amino acids in whey protein assist with fixing skin and tissues from wounds or medical procedure.

Weight gain and dietary lift: Individuals who need to put on weight can profit from whey protein. It's likewise useful on the off chance that an individual has a drawn out sickness and needs additional nourishment. "In the event that you can't get sufficient protein from entire food sources, a whey protein supplement can help," says Smith. "It's gainful for individuals who have biting or gulping problems or an absence of craving."

Aftereffects and dangers of whey protein

Whey protein is by and large safe for a great many people to take, as long as they don't have a dairy sensitivity. However, there are a few disadvantages:

Calorie content: Whey protein might be low fat and low carb, however it actually has calories. "An excessive number of calories from anything, including protein, prompts weight gain," Smith makes sense of.

Additional sugar or handled fixings: Numerous protein powders and shakes contain handled fixings like fake flavors, sugars or added sugar. "It's smarter to get your protein from entire food sources and a fluctuated diet, as opposed to an enhancement, bars or shakes," says Smith. "Assuming that you utilize an enhancement, search for one that rundowns whey protein as the main fixing."

Potential toxins: Protein supplements don't have severe guidelines like food varieties and medications. "The virtue probably won't be demonstrated in some protein supplements," says Smith. "They can have fillers or weighty metal toxins that aren't recorded on the name." Pick whey protein items that are NSF Confirmed for Game or affirmed by Informed Decision. These items have been autonomously tried for virtue.

Conceivable stomach related issues: Certain individuals experience clogging, the runs or sickness from taking whey protein, particularly assuming that they take enormous sums.

Whey protein has its place assuming you're a competitor building muscle or attempting to fill a few dietary holes. Yet, the vast majority as of now gets sufficient protein and don't require supplements.

"Your body can utilize 20 to 40 grams of protein at an at once. "Regardless of whether you're attempting to build up, taking sums higher than this isn't useful. The vast majority don't require whey protein to meet their protein prerequisites in the event that they're eating a solid eating routine."

Similarly as with any enhancement, it's ideal to talk about with your doctor before you begin taking protein supplements. They can impede a few meds or may really be hurtful for individuals with specific circumstances.

Red, bothersome skin (dermatitis). Research shows that babies who consume whey protein by mouth during the initial 3 a year of life have a lower chance of creating red, bothersome skin by the age of 3 years.

Inclined sensitivities and unfavorably susceptible responses (atopic sickness). Research shows that newborn children who consume whey protein by mouth during the initial 3 a year of life are less inclined to be inclined to sensitivities and unfavorably susceptible responses contrasted with babies who get standard recipe. Be that as it may, taking why protein probably won't be useful for treating atopic sicknesses once they create.

Weight reduction in individuals with HIV/Helps. Some exploration demonstrates the way that taking whey protein by mouth can assist with diminishing weight reduction in individuals with HIV.

Red, layered skin (psoriasis). Some proof shows that taking a particular whey protein remove (Dermylex Advantech Inc.) day to day for quite a long time can diminish psoriasis side effects.

Lung illness called constant obstructive aspiratory infection (COPD). Taking a particular whey protein supplement (Empower) every day for a very long time can further develop windedness yet not lung capability or personal satisfaction in individuals with COPD. Other exploration recommends that taking whey protein supplements doesn't further develop lung capability, muscle capability, or exercise resilience in individuals with COPD.

Osteoporosis. Research recommends that taking a beverage containing whey protein day to day for a considerable length of time doesn't work on bone thickness in that frame of mind with osteoporosis.

Weight reduction. Most examination recommends that taking whey protein alone, alongside diet changes, or while following an activity plan doesn't appear to decrease weight for overweight and large grown-ups. Be that as it may, whey protein could further develop body piece in overweight grown-ups when utilized alongside a changed eating routine. In overweight youngsters, drinking a whey protein refreshment for a considerable length of time appears to expand weight and weight file (BMI).

Inadequate Proof to Rate Viability for...

Athletic execution. Some clinical examination shows that taking whey protein in mix with strength preparing increments fit weight, strength, and muscle size. In any case, other exploration recommends no impact of whey protein on strength or bulk. Taking whey protein appears to further develop recuperation from practice better compared to starch supplements in undeveloped yet not prepared competitors.

Asthma. Early examination recommends that taking a particular sort of whey protein (HMS 90 Immunofec, Inc) every day for 30 days doesn't further develop lung capability in kids with asthma.

Disease. There is some proof that taking whey protein could assist with decreasing growth size in certain individuals with disease that has spread.

Cystic fibrosis. Early examination recommends that taking whey protein day to day for 28 days further develops lung capability in youngsters, yet not grown-ups with cystic fibrosis

Asthma brought about by work out. Early exploration recommends that taking whey protein day to day for 10 days further develops lung capability in individuals with asthma brought about by work out.

Non-alcoholic liver illness (nonalcoholic steatohepatitis, NASH). Early examination proposes that taking whey protein day to day for quite some time can work on liver capability in patients with NASH.

Hepatitis. Early exploration recommends that taking a particular kind of whey protein (Immunocal) day to day for a very long time can work on liver capability in certain individuals with hepatitis B. Be that as it may, it doesn't seem to help individuals with hepatitis C.

HIV/Helps. Early examination proposes that taking whey protein for a considerable length of time doesn't work on resistant capability in youngsters with HIV.

Elevated cholesterol. Early examination recommends that taking whey protein day to day while partaking in obstruction preparing doesn't lessen cholesterol levels or muscle versus fat in overweight men with elevated cholesterol.

Hypertension. Early examination recommends that drinking refreshment that contains whey protein day to day for a long time doesn't bring down circulatory strain in individuals with hypertension. Notwithstanding, taking hydrolyzed whey protein every day for quite some time can decrease pulse

Contaminations created while in the clinic. Early exploration proposes that taking a particular whey protein supplement (Beneprotein) every day for as long as 28 days likewise affects the pace of medical clinic procured diseases as taking a mix of zinc, selenium, glutamine, and metoclopramide.

Acquired messes that cause mental and formative issues (mitochondrial myopathies). Early examination recommends that taking a whey protein supplement day to day for one month doesn't further develop muscle strength or personal satisfaction in individuals with mitochondrial sicknesses.

Ovarian pimples (Polycystic ovarian disorder). Early exploration proposes that taking an enhancement containing whey protein day to day for a very long time can decrease body weight, fat mass, and cholesterol in individuals with ovarian growths. Be that as it may, whey protein doesn't further develop glucose and appears to diminish high-thickness lipoprotein (HDL or "great") cholesterol.

Throbbing and solidness brought about by irritation (polymyalgia rheumatica). Taking whey protein in a dairy item two times day to day for quite a long time doesn't further develop muscle capability, strolling speed, or other development tests in individuals with polymyalgia rheumatica.

Types

There are three essential kinds of whey protein; whey protein concentrate (WPC), whey protein disconnect (WPI), and whey protein Hydrolysate (WPH).

Whey protein concentrate - WPC contains low degrees of fat and low degrees of starches. The level of protein in WPC really relies on how concentrated it is. Lower end concentrates will more often than not have 30% protein and better quality up to 90 percent.

Whey protein segregate - WPIs are additionally handled to eliminate all the fat and lactose. WPI is ordinarily somewhere around 90% protein.

Whey protein hydrolysate - WPH is viewed as the "predigested" type of whey protein as it has proactively gone through halfway hydrolysis - an interaction essential for the body to retain protein.

WPH doesn't need as much absorption as the other two types of whey protein.

Additionally, WPH is generally utilized in clinical protein enhancements and baby equations in view of its better edibility and decreased allergen potential.

Muscle building and weight reduction

Whey protein supplementation alongside opposition exercise can assist with further developing muscle protein amalgamation and advance the development of lean tissue mass.

A review distributed in the Global Diary of Game Sustenance and Exercise Digestion presumed that "whey protein supplementation during obstruction preparing offers some advantage contrasted with opposition preparing alone." likewise, "guys who enhanced with whey protein had a more prominent relative increase in lean tissue mass."

Much better acquires in strength are related with whey disengage supplementation contrasted and casein.

This was shown in one more review distributed in the Worldwide Diary of Game Sustenance and Exercise Digestion, which reasoned that in "two gatherings of coordinated, opposition prepared guys whey separate gave fundamentally more noteworthy increases in strength, lean weight, and a diminishing in fat mass contrasted and supplementation with casein during a serious 10-week obstruction preparing program."

Kinds of protein powder

There are a few unique kinds of protein powder. Whey is the most well-known protein supplement and the one that scientists have would in general zero in on, however it isn't the one to focus on. Normal kinds of protein powder include:

Whey: This water-solvent milk protein is well known among competitors. It is a finished protein, implying that it contains each of the amino acids that the human body expects from food. The body ingests whey protein rapidly and without any problem.

Casein: This kind of protein is wealthy in glutamine, an amino corrosive that might accelerate muscle recuperation after work out. Casein comes from dairy, making it inadmissible for veggie lovers and individuals with milk sensitivities. The body processes this protein all the more leisurely, so taking it at night might be ideal.

Soy: Soy protein is an astounding option in contrast to whey or casein for individuals who don't consume dairy. It additionally contains every one of the fundamental amino acids.

Pea: Many plant-based protein powders contain pea protein, which is a top notch option in contrast to soy- and dairy-based proteins. Pea protein is a decent wellspring of the amino corrosive arginine.

Hemp: Hemp seeds are finished proteins that additionally contain fundamental unsaturated fats. This settles on hemp a brilliant decision for veggie lovers or those with dairy or soy sensitivities.

Whey or serum proteins are dissolvable milk proteins addressing around 20% of absolute milk proteins. The β-lactoglobulin, α-lactalbumin, protease peptone, serum egg whites, and immunoglobulins arranged by overflow structure the cow-like whey proteins. They are accessible as a fixing as whey powder, whey protein concentrates, and whey protein segregates, essentially made from whey — a side-effect of cheddar industry. The extraordinary qualities of whey proteins like solvency over an extensive variety of pH, positive dietary profile regarding fundamental amino acids, various usefulness, and moderately minimal expense make them an optimal fixing in figuring out wide cluster of food items. This part examines the utilization of whey proteins as fixings in food sources, the logical strategies utilized for whey protein examination, the design of the significant whey proteins, useful properties of whey proteins, and further developing usefulness of whey proteins, future patterns, and hotspots for additional data regarding this matter.

Whey proteins are utilized as a crucial fixing in a wide assortment of newborn child recipes particularly for untimely babies attributable to the way that it contains a considerable lot of the parts found in human bosom milk (Solak and Associated, 2012). The baby recipes containing whey proteins are consequently viewed as the best choices to bosom taking care of. The expansion of LF (a significant whey protein part) to a taking care of recipe can expand the degrees of Bifid bacteria in bottle-took care of children, which diminishes the capability of creating atopic sickness for in danger babies with family ancestry, as well as worked on gastrointestinal resistance. Specific sorts of whey proteins-based newborn child equations have likewise been displayed to assist with diminishing crying on account of juvenile colic. Moreover, whey proteins are an amazing decision for the hopeful mother who needs an expanded measure of proteins. Pregnancy can expand the body's protein needs by up to 33% (Gupta et al., 2012), this expanded prerequisite can be really accomplished in view of an eating regimen including whey proteins.

Whey proteins are important as elements for their useful and dietary perspectives; however flavor is a significant driver in the acknowledgment of whey protein fixings. Understanding the flavor credits of whey items is fundamental for the proceeded with outcome of the whey business. In a perfect world whey protein fixings ought to be flavorless, as this considers the best flexibility in fixing applications. Notwithstanding, off-flavors effectively foster in whey protein items because of lipid oxidation, proteolysis, and Mallard responses. These flavors start to foster in liquid milk, being impacted by the creature's eating regimen and milk taking care of. They likewise foster in whey during unit tasks in whey handling, fixing production, and capacity. There has been a lot of exploration in regards to the kind of whey protein fixings; but the maximum capacity of whey protein fixings might be acknowledged through proceeded with research on flavor decrease.

Whey protein is the water period of milk, whenever casein has been taken out. Its flavor is for the most part identical to that of meat and it additionally matches the light shade of poultry meat well. The capacity of whey protein to gel and the temperature at which this happens are to a still up in the air by temperatures applied during assembling of the whey protein itself (for ideal gelling, the assembling temperatures ought to be kept low). Gelling of a whey protein likewise relies upon pH levels and the grouping of salt inside a meat item. Most normally, whey protein concentrates of around 35% protein are utilized in meat items. Whey protein concentrates are not difficult to use in that frame of mind as they are profoundly solvent, with low thickness simultaneously.

The WBC of whey protein is somewhat low, yet its gelling limit is high. Whey protein is likewise in all actuality stable against changing pH values in meat items.

Whey protein fixings have become progressively significant in formed food sources throughout recent years. Whey proteins are generally provided as whey protein concentrates (80% protein) and whey protein confines (90% protein). Whey proteins are a side-effect from handling of other dairy items, outstandingly cheddar and casein, and consideration should be paid to the beginning of the whey as this influences both protein structure and mineral organization of the fixing. Whey proteins are significant healthfully as a balancer for different proteins in unambiguous nourishing applications, like baby formulae, and all alone as a rich wellspring of extended chain amino acids, significant in muscle sustenance. Whey proteins additionally have significant utilitarian advantages, especially as a result of their gelling and water-restricting limit, and furthermore due to their capacity to balance out interfaces in froths and emulsions. A scope of new innovations right now being investigated may lead to a scope of novel whey protein fixings with improved usefulness; notwithstanding, the drawn out maintainability of whey proteins as food fixings involves concern.

Polyacrylamide gel electrophoresis of whey proteins was first performed to measure the singular parts (Dear and Butcher, 1965). The partition and staining strategies were normalized and during every electrophoresis run a standard protein arrangement of whey proteins was likewise isolated and stained under similar circumstances as the test materials. In this manner the standard arrangements were exposed to similar treatment as the test arrangements. Densitometry examining of the stained protein containing gels followed by top region judgments was completed. By correlation with standard pinnacle regions individual protein centralizations of the test not entirely set in stone.

This part initially characterizes the expression "whey proteins" in accordance with the items in this book. We characterize whey proteins as the proteins not related with the casein micelle or other milk particles, for example, layer structures and physical and microbial cells. This section isolates the whey proteins into two classifications of major and minor whey proteins. The significant whey proteins talked about here are β-lactoglobulin, α-lactalbumin, serum egg whites, and immunoglobulins. A few qualities of these proteins are examined remembering their overflow for milk of different species, amino corrosive creation and sub-atomic construction, hereditary polymorphism, natural and innovative capability as well as their importance. The minor whey proteins remembered for this section are lactoferrin, proteose peptone 3, osteopontin, glycomacropeptide, lactoperoxidase, lysozyme, cathepsin D, corrosive phosphatase, and ribonucleases. As well as talking about the overflow, attributes and meaning of these minor whey proteins, this section sums up their significant highlights in a few helpful tables.

Some whey protein concentrates can go about as immunostimulatory and anticancer dietary parts when conveyed as a significant protein source to creatures and individuals. In a review, Rutherfurd-Markwick et al. (2005) researched the impacts of a known immunostimulatory WPC (IMUCARE), when given to mice in a changed milk powder (MMP), that was healthfully adjusted for small kids (matured one to three years).

Gatherings of BALB/c mice were taken care of with MMP-based eats less carbs regardless of IMUCARE WPC enhanced at 10.5 g/100 g of diet for times of about a month. Ex vivo immunologic measures demonstrated that splenic lymphoproliferative reactions, as well as blood and peritoneal leukocyte phagocytic movement, were raised in mice took care of MMP enhanced with IMUCARE WPC, in correlation with either mice took care of with MMP alone or to control mice that didn't get milk proteins. Conversely, both IMUCARE WPC-enhanced MMP and MMP alone were displayed to animate improved humoral resistance, with altogether raised serum and digestive system counter acting agent reactions to orally directed antigens being kept in these mice, contrasted and creatures took care of with no milk protein.

The outcomes affirm that IMUCARE WPC holds immunoenhancing viability when conveyed in a healthfully adjusted milk item and moreover distinguishes healthfully adjusted MMP as a potential immunostimulatory dietary food item. As well as supporting cell resistant capability, aftereffects of this work likewise demonstrate that both MMP and IMUCARE WPC-enhanced eats less carbs expanded immunoresponses in mice at both the foundational level (blood serum) and in the stomach mucosal climate (tests of digestive wash emissions).

Expulsion of Lipid from Whey and Whey Protein Parts

WPCs definitely contain levels of leftover lipid, disregarding endeavors by makers to eliminate however much as could be expected As would be normal, levels of remaining lipid increment with expanding protein fixation. Reports have proposed degrees of around 2.1% fat in 35% WPC, 3.7% fat in half WPC, and 7.2% fat in 80% WPC. As should be visible in the higher protein content items, the degree of lipid is very huge. Expulsion of the lipid from whey results in an improvement in ultrafiltration transition, yet in addition particularly further develops item usefulness. For instance, more elevated levels of lipid have been demonstrated to be unfavorable to the frothing and flavor attributes of WPC. Expulsion of lipids increments overwhelm whipping significantly, as well as expanding froth dependability. More significant levels of lipid likewise repress the intensity gelation properties of WPC.

The structure of the lipid part in WPC isn't like that of mass milk, being higher in phospholipid and milk fat globule film material.

In general, accordingly, the lipid part in whey is accepted to hinder a significant part of the possible usefulness of WPCs, and whey protein portions. The lipid portion in whey is additionally halfway answerable for the fouling of the layers on ultrafiltration handling of whey. Expulsion of the lipid division can hence further develop handling proficiency (on the off chance that ultrafiltration is utilized) as well as item usefulness.

Expulsion of such lipids from whey preceding ultrafiltration or fractionation can be accomplished by microfiltration utilizing layers of a suitable pore size to eliminate the nearly huge lipid-containing material. Be that as it may, fouling of microfiltration layers (apparently additionally by the lipid-containing division) in such cycles has, at this point, alleviated against broad business reception of this methodology. It is logical, notwithstanding, that upgrades in microfiltration layers combined with proper change of handling conditions will bring about expanded commercialization of such cycles sooner rather than later.

The expansion of calcium to total lipoproteins in whey has likewise been proposed as an option in contrast to microfiltration for lipid expulsion. While this cycle is in fact powerful, it might present specific troubles on increasing to business activity.

Some of the whey fractionation processes recently framed brings about the special exchange of any lipid-containing piece of the whey into one specific division. For instance, the lipid portion in whey is specially seen as in the part delivered by the Australian cycle using warm conglomeration. Such lipid material might be taken out from whey portions by, for instance, microfiltration. This would bring about a protein part with expanded usefulness, and a lipid division with brilliant emulsification qualities.

WPC contains lactose (to fluctuating degrees, contingent upon level of handling) and subsequently may not be reasonable for utilization by individuals who are lactose bigoted, nor is it appropriate for individuals who experience the ill effects of dairy milk protein sensitivities. Youngsters comprise a weak gathering for cow milk protein sensitivity, with 2%-7% fostering this sensitivity (Patel, 2015), and can prompt atopic dermatitis (skin inflammation). Be that as it may, enzymatically hydrolyzed WP might be better endured as they are less allergenic. Duane, Yang, Li, Zhao, and Huo (2014) showed that mice took care of with WPH had lower allergen city comparative with WPC. Nonetheless, the hydrolysis interaction creates harsh peptides which make the item less attractive. Despite the fact that ultrafiltration can be utilized to eliminate the bigger severe peptides this cycle will likewise bring about evacuation of possibly valuable peptides (e.g., bioactive peptides) and protein as well as making the item costlier.

An option for competitors who stay away from dairy items under any circumstance are the numerous accessible plant-based protein sources, albeit an enormous number contain lower levels of leonine (6%-8%) than creature based proteins (8%-11%) and hence may not invigorate MPS to a comparative degree as WP (Happiness et al., 2013). The most well-known plant-based protein source is soy protein as it is a greater protein than other vegetable proteins and SPI is the favored item type, as it contains the most elevated protein content at 90% (Paul, 2009). Various examinations did in obstruction prepared subjects have shown that supplementation with either SPI or WP accomplish comparative LBM gain (Paul, 2009). Rice protein separate has been displayed to help comparative changes in strength and body creation as WPI in obstruction preparing subjects (Satisfaction et al., 2013).

During assembling of whey protein concentrate (WPC) and whey protein separate (WPI) powders, careful steps are taken to guarantee ideal mechanical and healthful functionalities in regards to their end-use prerequisites. Be that as it may, the control of their stockpiling is still rather observational and primary and utilitarian changes happen, in spite of the monetary significance of these items. This section plans to give an outline of the exploration work in light of the stockpiling of WPC and WPI powders. It centers on the physicochemical changes at a molecule scale (e.g., microstructure, surface science) and a sub-atomic scale (e.g., protein-and lactose-related changes) happening during stockpiling as per the circumstances, remembering their effect for utilitarian properties (e.g., interfacial, frothing, emulsifying, and heat-instigated conglomeration properties). This part additionally features a few regions for development to limit the capacity instigated changes, for example, better observing of the Mallard response, following up on the key impacting factors, and foreseeing powders' changes.

Whey based fixings have a huge area of uses, including dairy items, dry mixes, wet mixes, arranged dry blends, newborn child food, soda pops/extraordinary dietary food varieties, sweets, handled meat, refreshments, frozen pastries, pastry kitchen items, spread details, and handled cheddar (Table 2). Whey fixings are additionally used to improve the tangible properties and they might be utilized as oil specialists in food varieties (Di Cicco et al., 2019; Hossain et al., 2020). The functionalities and utilizations of WPI/WPC can be additionally upgraded by changing the underlying conformity of the proteins. For example, pre-denatured whey protein totals have been found to work on the actual dependability of oil-in-water emulsions in cheddar and in basic liquid emulsion framework when whey fixings applied as emulsifying specialist (Çakır-Fuller, 2015; Li et al., 2020). The pre-treatment with warming possibly sets off incomplete or complete unfurling of the globular protein's tertiary adaptation and uncovered the secret hydrophobic amino gatherings, in this manner, expanding the extra volume and adaptability. Despite the fact that intensity actuated and additionally salt prompted (Ca2+) whey protein totals have exhibited remarkable functionalities as far as settling emulsion frameworks, modifying absorption energy of the exemplified oil in the emulsion drops, it is essential to call attention to that whey protein totals might bring about unreasonable turbidity, stage detachment, expanded thickness, gelation, and precipitation depending protein fixation, physicochemical circumstances and other natural/outward factors (Guo, 2019; Streicher et al., 2020).

Review have demonstrated the way that MWP can be a potential fat replacer in calorie thick food varieties, for example, meat, frankfurters, cheddar and quick food varieties by diminishing how much fat utilized and debilitating the level of lipid processing into the small digestive system (Kumar et al., 2018; Guo, 2019; Streicher et al., 2020). MWP is regularly utilized in the development of drinks, yogurt, frozen yogurt, cheddar, aged dairy items, dressings, and sauces (Guo, 2019). MWP in yogurt works on the rheological and tangible properties, especially smoothness in diminished fat and plain blended yogurt when contrasted with the full fat yogurt (Hossain et al., 2020). Size of the MWP altogether affects the rheological and tactile properties of the food items. For example, a microgel with a molecule size of lower than 10 μm, further develops smoothness and delicacy to yogurt and frozen yogurt among other day to day items; On the other hand, bigger molecule size might prompt a coarse and sandy mouthfeel (Dickinson, 2015; Hossain et al., 2020). MWP likewise upgrades the solidness of nutraceutical-stacked oil-in-water emulsion and holds the quality ascribes during openness to warm (Guo, 2019).

Cheddar Whey

Cheddar whey is a fluid gotten after the precipitation of milk casein in the cheddar making process, it is vital in the dairy business because of the enormous volume produced and its dietary sythesis. Around 90% of the volume utilized for cheddar creation is changed over completely to whey, which holds roughly 55% of the supplements contained in milk (Dragone et al., 2009). Among the supplements found in the cheddar whey, the biggest part relates to lactose 39-60 kg/m3, protein and mineral salts, 6-8 kg/m3, lipids 4-5 kg/m3, and dry concentrate 8%-10% (Dragone et al., 2011). These boundaries make cheddar whey a significant item with applications in the food and drug businesses. Nonetheless, the attributes of cheddar whey will rely upon the nature of milk, creature, breed, creature feed, wellbeing, lactation, and among different variables (Prazeres et al., 2012).

Every year on the planet is delivered around 24,000,000 tons of cheddar, which will bring about roughly 21,600,000 tons of cheddar whey. Because of the great organic oxygen interest (Body) of cheddar whey brought about by the high centralization of lactose, this result turns into a significant natural issue of dairy industry, and can be multiple times more dirtying than homegrown sewage. To follow natural regulation, in regards to the erroneous removal of cheddar whey, the businesses have been searching for options for its reuse. Most enterprises have been utilizing cheddar whey, and transforming it into whey powder, whey protein concentrates, lactose, and blended drink, for example, aged milk added of cheddar whey. Another choice is the utilization of fermentative cycles to acquire esteem added items, like unicellular proteins, alcohols (ethanol and butanol), nutrients, natural acids (lactic corrosive, succinic, and propionic corrosive), among others (Mollea et al., 2013; Dragone et al., 2009). In these items, the concentrated cheddar whey is all the more every now and again utilized because of its high supplements and lactose content, which, on account of maturation, helps the microbial development.

Cheddar whey is a huge result gotten from cheddar fabricating processes and its accessibility is becoming around the world. Whey was generally released because of its high Body (natural oxygen interest) and

COD (compound oxygen interest) values which fundamentally influence as an ecological toxin (Carvalho, Prazeres, and Rivas, 2013; A long while back, whey was utilized for creature taking care of and shower water system of fields. Biomass, metabolites and explicit particles may likewise be acquired through aging or synthetic response of whey. Somewhat recently, and because of the great added worth of certain parts, for example, whey protein and lactose, there has been an expansion in the utilization of cycles in light of convergence of whey by vanishing and fractionation into explicit parts utilizing centrifugation, particle trade or film filtration, permitting change of whey in exceptionally important items.

Different items can be acquired from handled whey, that is whey protein concentrate (WPC), detach (WPI) or hydrolysate (WPH), micro articulated whey protein, whey cream, whey powder (Yama et al., 2015). Specifically, whey protein is utilized as an added substance in a wide assortment of food, for instance cereals, nourishing enhancements, newborn child formulae, refreshments and dairy items, because of the expansion in the yield and improvement of healthful/mechanical qualities of the end results (Ipsen, 2017; Masotti, Cattaneo, Stuknytė, and De Noni, 2017; Wherry, Barbano, and Drake, 2019). Nonetheless, it is urgent to guarantee the shortfall of phage particles in these fixings in the event that they will be added before a maturation step to forestall phage contaminations (Geagea et al., 2015).

Cheddar whey might contain phage centralizations of up to 109 PFU/mL after cheddar fabricating. During its reusing interaction, whey cheddar is exposed to a warm treatment determined to dispense with waste microorganisms and the remanent BAL strains utilized as starter societies. This intensity therapy ought to be delicate to forestall protein denaturation (Atamer and Hinrichs, 2010; Geagea et al., 2015; Samtlebe et al., 2017). Despite the fact that dairy phages might be inactivated by warming, high thermostability of phage against warm medicines applied regularly to dairy process have been legitimate (Atamer et al., 2009; Briggiler Marcó et al., 2019; Capra et al., 2013; Geagea et al., 2015; Pujato et al., 2014; Wagner, Samtlebe, et al., 2017). As outcome, a high grouping of phages might stay infective after heat medicines. A while later, cheddar whey is exposed to focus (by dissipation as well as ultrafiltration), shower drying and various medicines relying upon the qualities of the ideal side-effects (Samtlebe, Wagner, Neve, et al., 2017). Specifically, the ultrafiltration interaction used to get WPC includes removed values running somewhere in the range of 20 and 40 kDa. Notwithstanding, milk protein and phages are held by ultrafiltration (film with a cut-off of 20 kDa) of skim milk. In this manner, these side-effects will be amassed in proteins yet additionally in phage particles, because of maintenance of the visions in the films (Samtlebe et al., 2015). During ultrafiltration step, whey might be concentrated up to multiple times, bringing about a protein grouping of roughly 4%. In this way, phage fixations as high as 109 PFU/mL in the whey might increment much more to reach 1010 PFU/mL after ultrafiltration (Atamer and Hinrichs, 2010).

Whey-Based Refreshments

Cheddar whey is a significant side-effect from the cheddar business, with a yield of 60-90 g/100 g corresponding to the all-out milk coagulated during the creation relying upon the cheddar type, addressing a huge wellspring of protein and energy. In the particular instance of goat cheddar whey created in Brazil, the most piece of goat cheddar make happens in little or medium-sized dairy plants and this result is frequently disposed of with next to no treatment as a profluent, turning into areas of strength for a. As another option, the utilization of cheddar whey in the creation of dairy drinks has been an exceptionally alluring choice, especially because of its healthy benefit (Buriti et al., 2014).

Whey contains 45%-half of complete milk strong, 70% of milk sugar (lactose), 20% of milk protein, 70%-90% of milk minerals, and practically every one of the water dissolvable nutrients present in the milk. The protein present in the whey contains around half ß-lactoglobulin, 25% of α-lactalbumin and 25% different proteins. Whey is the wellspring of calcium, phosphorus, and fundamental amino acids. The presence of this multitude of fixings makes whey a profoundly nutritious item (Devi et al., 2017).

In spite of the fact that, whey proteins have numerous characteristics which are viewed as sound, one of its primary proteins β-lactoglobulin (BLG) is the principal allergen of milk. LAB, microorganisms profoundly utilized in the elaboration of aged milk items can hydrolyze milk proteins and also, some of them can disintegrate BLG during development in whey and milk. Furthermore, types of L. acidophilus, L. paracasei, and Bifidobacterium not set in stone to breakdown the BLG allergenic epitopes in vitro (Wagoner and Foregeding, 2017; Pescuma et al., 2010).

Current customers can acknowledge a refreshment that has in any event a portion of the principal properties, for example, achievement positive high tangible quality, ability to revitalize, ideal financial cost, and great 'wellbeing picture'. With the distinctive properties of the whey flavor hindering with different seasoning fixings and the handling costs adding to the quickly rising worth of the waste, the eventual fate of the whey beverages might lie fundamentally in the last property, the extraordinary nutraceutical standards of the some whey parts. Customer inclinations like comfort, flavor, and practicability, dietary benefit, and options accessible are for the most part influencing the market development of the utilitarian beverages (Chavan et al., 2015).

In a whey refreshment study, lower lactose debasement is seen during the creation of the cheddar whey based drinks, in correlation with delivered matured milk by conventional development of kefir grains. No huge contrasts are found between the examples toward the finish of the maturations while with respect to lactic corrosive and acidic corrosive sums, pH values and last ethanol fixations, as well as primary unstable development. It is accounted for that cheddar whey and deproteinized cheddar whey can be utilized as the substrates for the creation of kefir like beverages like aged milk kefir (Magalhães et al., 2011).

In an alternate report high contamination dairy industry squander ricotta cheddar whey changed into a fixing in the development of a synbiotic matured dairy drink, enhancing this waste and diminishing how much cheddar whey joined into the dairy wastewater. The outcomes show that dairy savor creation this study is gathered as probiotic and prebiotic as indicated by Brazilian regulation (Schlitz et al., 2015).

Aged whey drinks have low thickness, gentle flavor and low reasonability of probiotic microorganisms whenever contrasted and matured milk items. Hence, it requires utilizing sufficient expansion of starter societies and fixings might build these properties of the last item. There are many investigations about expansion of a few natural product juices and parts to the whey-based matured drinks. In Bulatovic et al. (2014) research a probiotic strain Lactobacillus rhamnosus ATCC 7469, ABY-6 starter culture and milk (30% v/v) added substances' consequences for the quality rules of matured whey-based refreshment are examined. It is showed that whey-based refreshment has advantageous surface and sensorial models like customary items. enough tactile properties and has a time span of usability of least 20 days. In another review, Sabokbar and Khodaiyan (2015) have assessed pomegranate juice and whey blend matured with kefir grains as original probiotic refreshment. Pomegranate juice and whey blend is found a legitimate substrate for the creation of probiotic dairy-natural product juice refreshment by kefir grains and the tangible properties of the beverage. Organic product drinks contain modest quantity of protein as a wholesome component. Fortress of natural product drinks with protein is a troublesome issue because of protein security in acidic and ionic circumstances. In a connected report, prepared to-serve (RTS) mango refreshment is sustained with changed whey protein and its quality properties are considered. Whey protein is hydrolyzed with papain to foster its strength in acidic circumstances. The water holding capability of whey protein expanded twice after the hydrolysis. Whey protein is added at 2%, 3%, and 4% (w/v) levels for stronghold of drink mango RTS. Stream conduct of the drink isn't impacted with the expansion of hydrolyzed whey protein at every one of the levels, altogether. The mango drink with hydrolyzed whey protein (3% w/v) is seen as satisfactory with high tangible imprints and dependability during warm handling and stockpiling in glass bottles (Yadav et al., 2016).

In other comparable review antioxidative and antimicrobial exercises of whey-based matured soy drinks with curcumin supplementation are assessed. Soy milk is ready by adding whey in water and curcumin. Maturation is directed by Str. thermophilus

NCDC323 (ST323) and L. acidophilus NCDC 195 (LA195) lactic societies. It is accounted for that LA195 and ST323 at various degrees of curcumin showed antimicrobial impact against E. coli, B. cereus, S. aureus, L. monocytogenes, Shigella dysenteriae, and Salmonella typhi with hindrance zone somewhere in the range of 16 and 23 mm. Greatest cell reinforcement action (989.70 TEAC (mu M)) can be gotten by the combination of LA195 + ST323 with curcumin. As per 9-point Decadent scale, soy drink with 12% sugar arrangement is taking high scores concerning variety and flavor. Item is steady for 4 days at 4°C. Cancer prevention agent movement (TEAC) diminished from 986.46 to 702.58 µM on the fourteenth day of capacity.